TAKING CARE OF THE CAREGIVER

BY

CHRISTINE RENEE

HAR Publishing, LLC

USA

Contents

Preface

This book is for all the many caregivers around the world working from home, in group homes, individual person's home (home health care), hospitals, assisted living, elder care facilities, nursing homes, etc... You are in demand and the work you do can be demanding. It's important to remember as a primary caregiver you are a hero but not a superhero.

Being a caregiver is a good work. However, there are many day-to-day challenges that one must consider before becoming a caregiver. And many are without any formal training and or knowledge of the good, the bad, and difficulties that comes along with administering care. Even those with formal training, you'll find this book to serve as a reminder and encouragement to your overall health and well-being

In order to prevent fatigue, burn out, and personal illnesses that comes from exhaustion. Every caregiver must learn how to take care of themselves *first* without feeling guilty or selfish in doing so. Your health is just as important and the ones you care for.

The information you obtain throughout this book will help you manage time and understand, caregivers all around the world that are going through similar situations.

This book is full of practical information on how to recognize and avoid anxiety, fatigue, burnout, and how to seek outside resources and help. Use this book for instruction and examples on how to take care of yourself as you care for others. It is only when we first help ourselves can we effectively help others

Acknowledgments

I would like to acknowledge God for all the many gifts and talents He has bestowed upon me, one of which is *caregiver*. Also like to thank my mother for allowing me to take care of her during this season of her life. It hasn't been an easy journey. However, it has been an honor and a privilege taking care of her while take care of myself as well. I have learned more about myself on another level in this season. Even with all the years of training that I have had, there have been many days I felt overwhelmed and frustrated. But I made a firm decision to hang in there and take care of her myself.

I like to also acknowledge Mike for inspiring me to get into nursing. Over two decades ago, he was the one who planted the seed that I should become a nurse. Although I never finished obtaining a degree in nursing. The advice he gave me years ago has been an integral part of my destiny. I like to acknowledge all the many nursing schools (several of which I attended), instructors, organizations, hospitals, nursing homes, and care giving facilities and agencies that I have attended and worked for over the years. All the many instructions that I have received over the years have inspired me to become one of the *best* caregivers I know how to be. I have cared for hundreds if not thousands of people, young and old. I have worked with people from all walks of life. I have cared for family members as well, and it has been a wonderful journey.

Special thanks to all caregivers around the world! Thank you for all you do. It takes an incredibly special person to serve others in their time of need.

This book is dedicated to my paternal grandmother who is no longer with us. She was the first person in my family I had the honor and the privilege to visit and care for on many occasions. I miss her dearly!

Introduction

It's morning and I'm sitting at the kitchen table feeding my mother her breakfast. In between feedings, I'm *typing* the introduction to this book. I like to multitask. It's something I do often since becoming mom's fulltime caregiver. Taking care of her hasn't been easy for me, emotionally and physically. However, I love what I do. I take care of her fulltime and we live together. Therefore, my *job* as a caregiver is 24 hours a day, and seven days a week.

My mother was diagnosed with dementia several years ago. And since I have a nursing background, I became her primary caregiver. I take care of all her physical needs, such as bathing, incontinence care, cooking, feeding, laundry, hair, nails, mouth care, medication administration, medical appointments, etc... I'm also an ordained minister, therefore, I make sure she is spiritually cared for as well.

I have over 20 years' experience as a caregiver. I have had the opportunity to care for people in hospitals, nursing homes, and private duty homes for decades. I take pride in what I do.

Taking care of my mother has truly been a journey. Not just a journey from the perspective of administering care and making sure all her needs are met. The journey has been more than just caring. It has been one of humongous sacrifice and responsibility. It has also been an honor and a privilege. I believe God has called me to be a caregiver. And although, I thought I was going to become a registered nurse. God had another plan.

Somedays my mother doesn't even remember who I am. She thinks, she lives in a nursing home and I'm just one of the caregivers or nurses, caring for her. Nevertheless, I work hard each and every day to make her comfortable, peaceful, happy, and content. She's seventy-six at the time of the writing this book and my prayer is she lives a long and blessed life.

Being a caregiver doesn't come without its challenges. Inside the home or whether working outside the home. Taking care of another is a task. Be it children, spouse, parent, friend or significant other. Caregiving is work and it is a job.

Over the years I have worked with an array of clients. As I've mentioned I worked in hospitals with adults and children. Home health care with incapacitated adults. However, most of my caregiving experience has been with the elderly population (geriatric care). I can truly say I enjoy administering care to the elderly. Over the years I have met some of the most wonderful people, from different backgrounds, ethnicities, and social economic variations.

People are aging and living longer. Most will need assistance with their physical, mental, and spiritual care before leaving this earth. However, in most cases many caregivers may or may not understand how essential it is to take proper care of themselves. Many lose focus when it comes to their wellbeing. Especially when the care they are giving is for a loved one. A *good* caregiver is always trying to give the best care in order to ensure the one they are caring for is well taken care of.

In reality caregivers must learn to *live* their best life while caring for others and recognize symptoms of burnout and fatigue. If not, sooner or later they'll find selves needing someone to care for them. Although it may appear domestically an easy "job" in the eyes of outsiders. Being a caregiver can be very demanding. Especially when you are taking care of one or multiple people who are mentally and or physically incapacitated. The pull on one can be enormous.

As with any job burnout is a key element one must manage mentally and physically. Therefore, caregivers must learn to take time to relax, and do things for themselves *daily*. Practicing self-care, relaxation, meditation, and spiritual applications is what this book is really all about. Caregivers must put into practice daily selfcare. And consider their health as well. They must also renew their minds and meditate on things that are positive, noble, reputable, authentic, compelling, gracious, the best, and beautiful.

Most importantly be happy, eat healthy, and always be mindful of their overall mental, spiritual, and physical health.

If caregivers learn to put some of the things discussed throughout each chapter in this book into practice daily, on a consistent basis. They'll have a better chance at being a healthier and happier caregiver. Take note! Everything in life can work together for the good. If it is Gods divine purpose that we care for others. Then He will make sure when it is our turn to receive care it will come back in return.

Learn to discern the difference between excess baggage and clutter in your life and try to eliminate them immediately. Also learn that people can be a blessing or an hinderance to your overall health and progress. This is not to say the client, person, or patient you are caring for is a hinderance. It can very well be anybody that is *not* helping you to do your job as a caregiver effectively or better. You may have to consider what is best as it pertains to relationships that cause unnecessary stress.

God and scripture are mentioned throughout this book. Because God honors caregivers. Jesus Himself was a servant and cares for humanity. He was concerned about the well-being of people. Therefore, excel in harmony, peace, joy, and happiness. And consider journaling on the pages provided throughout this book. Take notes about yourself and make changes in your life if necessary, that will be beneficial and good for your overall wellbeing.

Stay focused and keep in mind, most people are *not* gifted nor afforded the honor and privilege such as yourself to be a caregiver. Some may never understand nor appreciate the acts of service you render in caring for others. Some will even consider your work meager, lazy, or demeaning. Others may judge your motives. Nevertheless, stay focused because God knows how hard it is to give up your life goals to serve another. He knows your heart and He is a rewarder to those who do good. He sees all and He knows all.

Most of all don't become negative, angry, bitter, or at odds with yourself and others. And stop worrying and fretting. Enjoy your job and your life. Learn to live, love, laugh, and enjoy the journey as much as you can. Joy is where your strength comes from and as a caregiver you are going to need a lot of strength on a daily basis.

Note: The enemy of your soul would love for you to go hard and burnout! Therefore, Pace yourself and set boundaries so you can fulfill your calling and enjoy caring for yourself and others with excellence!

CHAPTER I
WHO AND WHAT IS A CAREGIVER?

Most caregivers are family members, spouses, adult children, parents of small children, friends, love ones, or professionals working in hospitals, nursing homes, or some aspect of health care. Caregivers are the ones who are able to care for and make decisions for individuals with mental and or physical disabilities.

Most caregivers have never been to nursing school, registered, licensed, nor certified to be a caregiver. However, they administer care, medications, clean, cook, and look after those who can't care for themselves. They're not a nurse. But many can teach some nurses a thing or two. When it comes to taking care of a sick incapacitated individual, caregivers are at their best. It's amazing how caregivers care for others and the many things that do.

As baby boomers age and grow older the more this population will need some type of assistance. From womb to tomb, everyone at some point has or will need some type of care. Whether caring for someone in your family or outside the family.

Anyone can be a caregiver. Whether male or female caring for someone who needs assistance is a job. Here's a list and various categories in which caregivers can fall in:

- Husband, wife -administering spousal care.
- Grown children -administering care to elderly parents.
- Relative -administering care to another relative.
- Home Health Aide
- Group Home Assistance and Coordinators
- Friend -administering care to a friend.
- Hospital Personal Caregivers (Registered Nurse, Certified Nurse, Licensed Nurse, etc.) - administering care to patients within a hospital setting.
- Nursing Home Caregivers (RN, CNA, LPN, etc.) - administering care to residence within a nursing facility.
- Parents administering care to sick a child or taking care of their own children in general.
- Hospice Nursing and Nurse Assistants
- Patient Advocates
- Assisted Living and Elderly Care
- Continuum of Care Facilities

- Dementia Care (Alzheimer's) Facilities

No matter what category you're in. Being a caregiver is demanding and can be over whelming at times. Feelings of being over-worked can be startling. However, from this day forward if you haven't already, ...consider yourself *blessed*. Blessed to be a blessing. Nothing is more rewarding than being able to give back to those who need help with daily living. Don't grow weary in doing good. Because at the appointed time you will reap a harvest of good if you don't quit. God will reward you for your faithfulness serving others.

There is a saying you reap what you sow. You get back what you give out, whether good or bad. However, nothing is more imperative as you care for others, that you take good care of yourself. Because if your health and wellbeing is not up to par, then you won't be any good to anyone else. You are a caregiver and you are needed, so take good care of yourself! Because without you those that need nurturing and care could possibly be left alone and face neglect.

"NOTES"

_____
_____
_____
_____
_____
_____
_____
_____
_____
_____
_____
_____
_____
_____
_____
_____
_____
_____
_____
_____
_____
_____
_____
_____
_____
_____

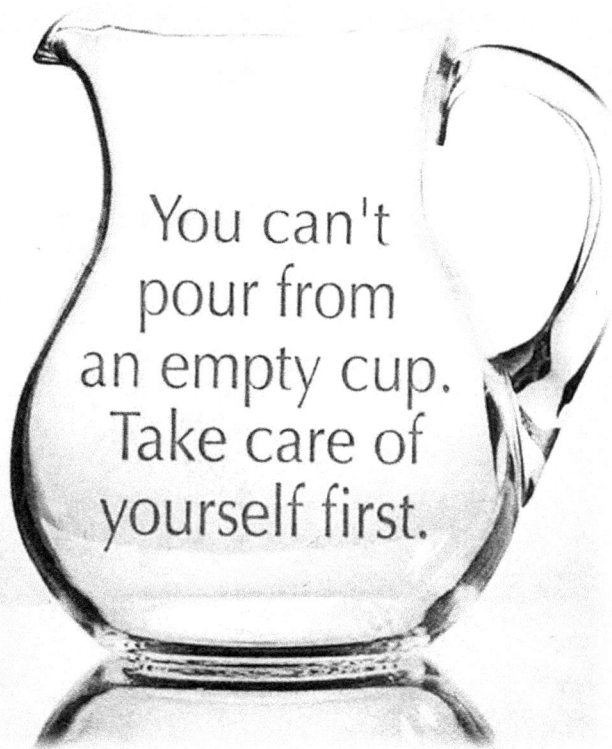

You can't
pour from
an empty cup.
Take care of
yourself first.

JOuRnAL HeRe.....................

Chapter II
Why Me?

Sometimes it's difficult being a caregiver. Feelings of being underrated and unappreciated has led many caregivers to asking ...why me? Why am I the one doing all the caring? Why am I the one to look after my aging parents? Why is my child, adult friend, spouse, or relative incapacitated or ill in this season of life of my life? Why me, has led many seeking and answers and feeling frustrated.

Many are raising children who need physical and or mental care beyond the scope of everyday parenting. Not to mention the stress that comes along with being a parent or single parent not having the necessary help when needed. Many have just finished raising children and getting them out the house and off to college. And all of the sudden they find themselves caring for an elderly parent. Some are caring for others on a fulltime basis with many considerations and responsibilities. Which they often find themselves unprepared and not ready for the task.

Whether you work from home or in a caregiving facility. You are the person *called* to get the job done. It's not the question of why me? But the situation warrants you to step up and be the caregiver in this season of your life. Let's face it somebody has to do it! And you may as well be to the one to administer care to those who aren't able to care for themselves. Therefore, learn to take care of yourself as well. Make it a priority of taking care of yourself before you care for anyone. You have to take care of yourself in order to be effective and proficient at what you do.

It's a job being a caregiver. But, it's a good work. Therefore, don't let anyone belittle you or put you down for the service you render. You are the one "called" to care for individuals in need. So, never forget you are needed.

Giving is one of the key words in caregiver. And sowing your life and time into another whether paid or not is a great place to be in.

Note: Stay focused and get rid of all clutter out of your life, so you can be a blessing. Don't look at your current situation as a burden. It's just a season you are in.

It's okay to ask why? I know for myself... I asked God many of time, "why now"? I never had children and I'm in the prime of my life. Why am I having to deal with so great a responsibility of taking care of my mother, in this season.

In the beginning when I first started taking care of my mother, I felt burdened and locked down, so to speak. I was used to living by myself and doing what I wanted to do, when I wanted to. So, you can image how difficult it was for me to give up everything. My job, home, lifestyle, and freedom.

If I would have dwelt on the why. I could have missed the opportunity of a lifetime being a blessing to her. No one can care for your love ones the way you can.

If we get in a rut of wondering why, then we can set ourselves up for failure. Which can lead to inevitably transitioning into a state of being depressed, remorseful, and down trodden. Or even worse we can become bitter, angry, and frustrated.

Remember this is just a season you are in and seasons change. Learn the lessons that are necessary to be learned in this season. And don't be so hard about the situation. Remember God will not forget your labor of love and you will reap a harvest of care that you have sown, if you don't quit and give up.

NOTE:

HANG IN THERE!

THINGS TO DO LIST

_____

_____

_____

_____

_____

_____

_____

_____

CHAPTER III
IS THIS A BURDEN, OR A GIFT?

Caregivers have an awesome responsibility. Taking care of anyone whether they're an adult, small child, sick child, etc.... Caregivers are called upon to provide a variety of assistance with activities of daily living (ADL's). The person receiving care usually needs help with activities of daily living such as feeding, bathing, toileting, dressing, housekeeping, and management of household responsibilities if they are unable to for themselves.

The emotional experiences involved in providing care can be overwhelming for the average person. Feelings of inadequacy can lead to anxiety, frustration, isolation, and exhaustion. All of which can lead one to feeling emotionally guilty and with regrets. The bottom-line is being a caregiver is no easy task. In some cases, the task can be a burden and gift at the same time.

Taking care of another can be a heavy load and responsibility. There will be times you will doubt that you can deliver the appropriate care. And there will be days you'll feel like quitting. But remember there is hope.

The burden of it all stems from the daily commitment and often times weariness that comes with caring for an individual who is unable to care for themselves. The gift is you're able to help others. Galatians 6:9 says, do not become weary in doing good, for in due season you will reap a harvest if you do not faint or give up (Holy Bible, paraphrased). You can't give up or quit. If you quit you may not reap a harvest of good tidings for yourself.

Note: The person you are caring for is dependent and depending upon you. However, while you are caring for others you mustn't jeopardize your own health in the process. If you have to reach out for help then by all means please do so.

Some of the challenges caregivers working from home deal with:

- Managing time. Caregivers often find they have less time for themselves and other family members.
- Emotional and physical stress.
- Lack of privacy.
- Financial strain.
- Sleep deprivation.
- Afraid to ask for help.
- Depression and isolation.

The importance of taking care of yourself first is best explained when flying on an airplane. The flight attendants always inform passengers... if the airplane cabin losses oxygen and the oxygen mask descend. The first thing you should do is put your oxygen mask on first before you assist anyone else with their mask. Only when you secure your mask first will you be effective enough to help others. Caring for yourself is the most important thing you can do as a caregiver. When your needs are met you and the person you are caring for benefits.

Taking responsibility for your own health is a never-ending process. The impact of a chronic or progressive illness; or a debilitating injury to someone that you are caring for can be a great strain. Therefore, you must take responsibility for your own personal well-being and make sure you get your needs met.

Many times, certain attitudes and beliefs stand in the way of self-care. However, not taking care of yourself can become a lifelong problem and pattern. A lifelong pattern where you feel like caring for others is a lot easier than caring for yourself. As a caregiver you must ask yourself, "what good will I be if I become ill, or what if I die"?

Breaking old patterns and habits as it relates to selfcare may not be easy, but it can be done. The first thing you must decide to do is remove all personal barriers and identify anything that may cause you to overlook yourself. Don't think you're being selfish if you put your needs *first*. And don't feel inadequate asking for help. You don't have to prove anything to anybody. Do the best you can. But not to the point of injuring yourself.

Sometimes caregivers have a misconception that increasing their workload will make it better for the one they are caring for. This can be misleading and can lead to additional stress and strain. Poor self-care can get in the way of providing excellent care.

Some of the most common questions and burdens caregivers have, are:

- If I don't do it, no one will.
- If I, do it right, I will get the love, attention, and respect I deserve. Our family always takes care of our own.
- I promised myself I would always take care of my parents.

Examples and barriers that can cause unnecessary anxiety are:

- Thinking you're the only one that is good at providing care.

- Thinking you can't rest during the day for a few minutes.

Don't forget the mind tends to believe what you tell it. And most caregivers tend to want to control what cannot be controlled. This often leads to feelings of failure, fatigue, and frustration. Which often leads to an inclination to ignoring one's own needs. Ask yourself what is getting in your way and keeping you from taking care of yourself. Once you identify any personal barriers and unnecessary burdens to good self-care. You can then begin to change your behavior and move forward one step at a time towards taking effective care of yourself, as you care for others.

Try to reduce personal stress and always factor in how you can adjust and cope with stressful situations or events that are inevitable. If you feel you can't handle a certain situation. The best result is to pause and walk away from the situation and evaluate what your perception is in the circumstances. Take note to whether you see the glass as half-full or half-empty, so to speak. And remember it's important that you seek counsel from trusted family members, friends, or a professional counselor who understands what intel's being a caregiver.

Levels of stress can be influenced by many factors, including:

- Whether your caregiving is voluntary or involuntary.
- If you feel you have no other choice in taking on the responsibilities, of being a primary caregiver. In this instance the chances are you will experience a greater level of stress, strain, and resentment.
- Your relationship with the care recipient. Sometimes people care for another with the hope of healing a relationship. If healing does not occur, you may feel regret and discouragement.
- Your coping abilities. How you coped with stress in the past predicts how you will cope now. Identify your current coping strengths so that you can build on them.
- Your caregiving situation. Some caregiving situations are more stressful than others. For example, caring for a person with dementia is often more stressful than caring for someone with a physical limitation.
- Whether or not support is available.

Recognize early signs of stress, which may include irritability, sleep problems, and forgetfulness. Know the warning signs and make changes as quickly as you can. Don't wait until you are overwhelmed.

Identify what you can and cannot change is important. And remember, you can only change yourself. You cannot change another person. When you try to change things which you have no control over, you only increase the level of frustration. Learn to take action to reduce stress. Versus trying to be in control. Stress reducers can be as simple as taking a daily walk and other forms of activities such as; gardening, meditation, or having coffee with a friend.

Note: Many caregivers don't know how to marshal the goodwill of others and many are reluctant to ask for help. Many don't want to admit that they can't handle everything by themselves.

Timing is important. A person who is tired and stressed might not be available to recognize when their emotions are controlling them. Our emotions are messages to which we need to listen to. They exist for a reason. However negative or painful, our feelings are useful tools for understanding what is happening to us, when we feel guilt, anger, and resentment contain important messages. Learn from them and take appropriate action.

Note: It may be time to seek treatment for depression especially if you are having thoughts of suicide. It is not selfish to focus on your physical health as well as your mental health.

Thinking about your needs is an important part of your job. You are responsible for your self-care. Therefore, focus on self-care practices such as:

- Learn and use stress-reduction techniques, like prayer, taking a walk, reading your bible.
- Attend to your healthcare needs.
- Get proper rest and diet.
- Exercise regularly, even if only for 10 minutes a day.
- Take time off without feeling guilty.
- Practice reading a good book or taking a warm bath to relax.
- Seek and accept the support of others.
- Seek supportive counseling when you need it, or talk to a trusted counselor, friend, or pastor.
- Identify and acknowledge your feelings.
- Change the negative ways you view situations.
- Set goals.

It's a blessing to be a servant and to serve others in need. If you have the "gift" of being a caregiver. Know your service is not in vain. Look at it as helping God administer His love and mercy through you to another. God is not going to forget your labor of love. The Bible says, whatsoever a man soweth that is what he or shall reap (Galatians 6:7).

Just think, how many caregivers have given up or put aside their life goals to care for another. Or put everything aside and on hold to go to nursing school, so they can give back to others. Or what about the person who hasn't gone to school but just somehow by the grace of God is able to be a caregiver to their children or incapacitated love one. What an awesome sacrifice.

Start looking at your role as a caregiver as a sacrificial responsibility, even if you don't get paid. Take the worry out of it and the feeling of being stuck in a situation that is a burden. Even though it may be hard and difficult at times. Everyday get up and start your day with something positive. Tell yourself, "I'm going to work in excellence and administer the best care I can today." Read the bible, say a prayer, make confessions and don't be lazy. Put your best foot forward and work with all your heart and soul. God will reward you as you sow seeds of mercy, grace, and love. It will come back to you. This concept has helped me to keep sowing good works so I can reap a harvest of care when it's my turn to be cared for!

NOTE: Don't Quit!

Reflections

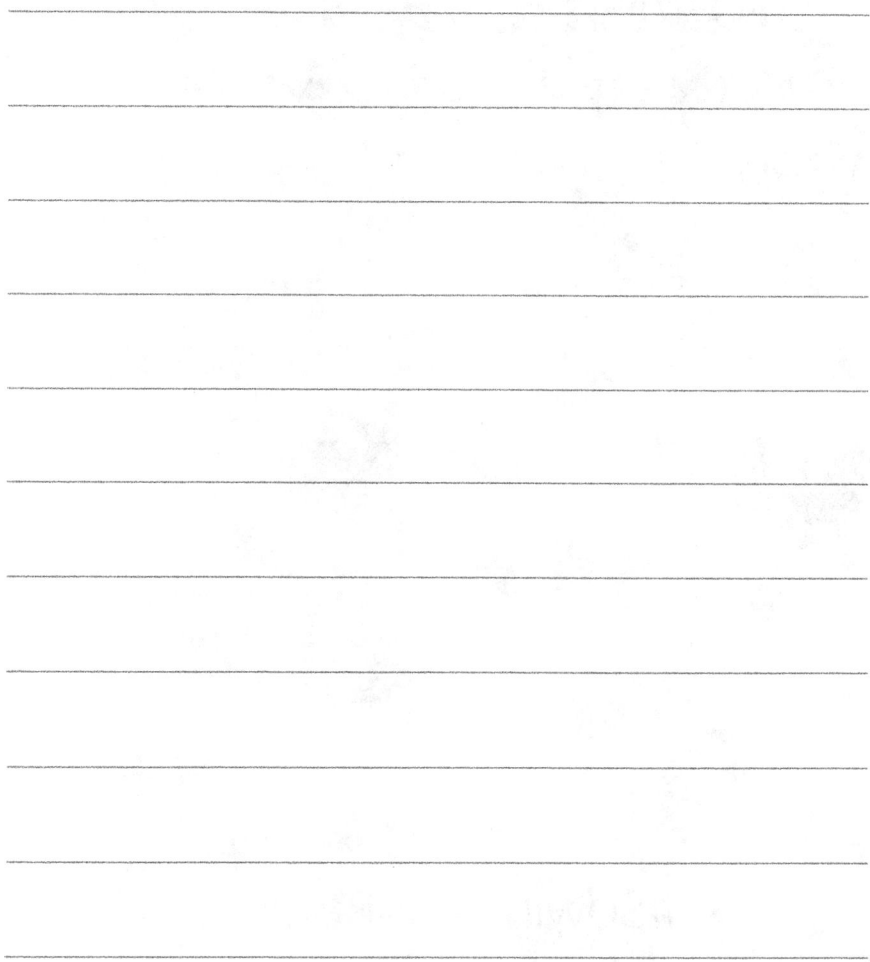

Remember: Sow good works and you'll reap a good harvest of care when it's your turn to be cared for!

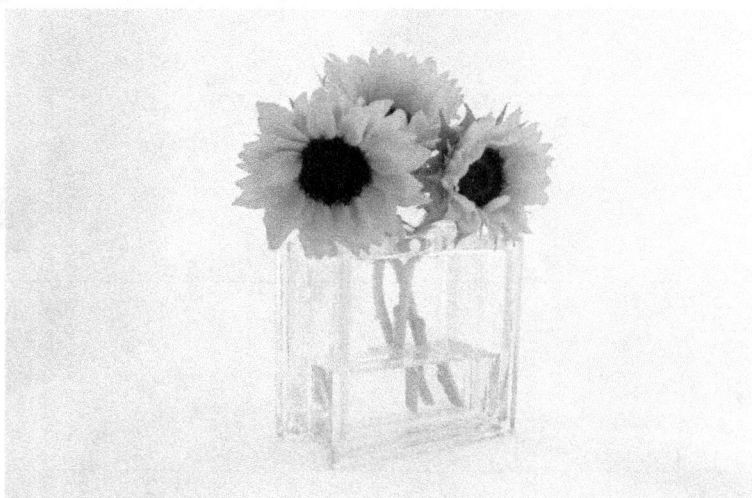

#SowingAndReaping

CHAPTER IV
DEALING WITH ANXIETY

Dealing with anxiety can be difficult from a caregiver's perspective. Adjusting to the people you care for and those with disease can often cause severe life changes. Therefore, when dealing with anxiety, one must recognize the symptoms of anxiety and learn to handle the symptoms. When it comes to a caregiver's individual's life, dealing with anxiety becomes vitally important for all involved.

I am not a medical doctor, however, there are signs and symptoms that comes with anxiety, such as irritability, restlessness, lack of concentration, racing thoughts, fatigue, excessive worry, fear, insomnia, nausea, palpitations, and trembling. Being a caregiver involves a range of emotions. If you find your emotions going reckless, you may need to make changes in your caregiving situation.

One on one care can be over whelming. For instance, when someone is diagnosed with Alzheimer's disease or suffering from some form of dementia. The sudden loss of control is incredibly frustrating to the person with dementia and incredibly worrisome to family members as well. No one wishes to find a loved one who is unsure of their surroundings or status in life.

Many individuals with dementia move in with family members or are cared for in centers that specializes in helping people with memory lost. Caregivers are needed to support them throughout the rest of their life.

Caregivers inside and outside of facilities, must remember everything has a season and anxiety doesn't have to be the norm. Especially with one-on-one care. Caregivers rendering care in the homes of people who need care must learn to embrace the season they are in.

Learn to embrace caring for yourself and other family members in this *season* is vitally important. And remember this to shall pass. Because with every activity under the heaven there is a season. Ecclesiastes 3 states, there is a time for everything:

a time to be born and a time to die,

a time to plant and a time to uproot,

a time to kill and a time to heal,

a time to tear down and a time to build,

a time to weep and a time to laugh,

a time to mourn and a time to dance,

a time to scatter stones and a time to gather them,

a time to embrace and a time to refrain from embracing,

a time to search and a time to give up,

a time to keep and a time to throw away,

a time to tear and a time to mend,

a time to be silent and a time to speak,

a time to love and a time to hate,

a time for war and a time for peace.

Even though there is great gain for all your labor of love. Don't let worry steal your joy and peace. And don't wear yourself out. I have personally experienced anxiety and the burden that comes with being a caregiver. I know the feeling of being worried and tired all too well. However, I refuse to quit and give up on caring for others and my mother, in this season of my life.

Sometimes the intentions of others are well meaning. However, for the most part caregivers are often left alone to sort out the logistics of who, what, when, how, and where by themselves. It's not that they don't won't or need help from others. But you may feel as though you must keep going and render the best care you know how, *alone*. Help is always good. But this depends on your personality. Whether you like working alone or with a group of people. The ultimate choice is yours.

Whatever you do learn to find at least one person you can count on. Even if it's just a friend that has an ear to hear your anxieties, your worries, your fears, and your frustrations. Being able to vent to someone you trust and someone that won't judge you or make assumptions. In most cases, this is all you need.

Make sure you get the proper "help" if needed so you can get plenty of rest. Because you are only *able* to finish your course as a caregiver with proper rest. Don't let pride or overt excellence; and being too picky cause you to not utilize resources and people who can help you. Take one day at a time. When you feel frustrated, take a break from the situation.

You may need to hire a sitter or home health aide to watch the one you are caring for in the event you have to get out from some of your duties as a caregiver. You may have to leave the one you are caring for with a trusted relative or friend while you take care of other things, such as, your personal things. Like your household business, your children, and spouse's needs. Remember this is just a season you are in. And seasons don't last forever.

Note: You may feel anxious and frustrated for have feelings that you want more out of life. You may even feel stuck and trapped. But take this season for what it is and realize things will eventually change.

In the meanwhile, study to be quiet and work diligently. Make sure you watch what you say about the ones you are caring for. And make sure you are careful what you say about yourself. For instance, you may feel tired and very well may be tired, but don't have to keep saying it or confessing it. Remind yourself daily, you can do all things through Christ who strengthens you (Philippian 4:13). Rest when you can and remember the joy of the Lord is your strength!

Communication is very important as a caregiver. Here are some guidelines to use when communicating your needs:

1. Respect the rights and feelings of others. Do not say something that will violate another person's rights or intentionally hurt them. Recognize that the other person has the right to express their feelings as well.

2. Be clear, specific, and speak directly to the person. Don't hint or hope the person will guess what you need. Other people are not mind readers. When you speak directly about what you need or feel, your chances of reaching understanding is greater.

3. Be a good listener. Listening is the most important aspect of any communication.

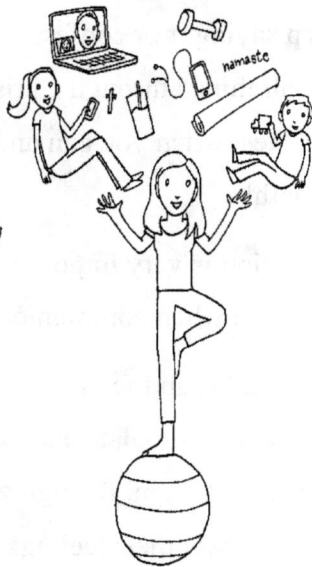

Balancing
Act

SET-UP A WEEKLY CALENDAR SO YOU CAN
LEARN TO BALANCE YOUR TIME

M	T	W	T	F	S	S

Having balance in every area of
your life is key to your success!

CHAPTER V
BALANCING YOUR TIME

Balancing time is of the essence when caring for another. Planning, prioritizing, organizing, and staying focused will help you to administer care more effectively and manage yourself at the same time. Balancing time is all inclusive to your health, finances, family, career, goals, and selfcare.

As a caregiver you are expected to do a good job even if you don't feel like it. But if you are out of balance, you will not be able to help anyone effectively. Therefore, give yourself grace to take breaks when possible. When practicing balance and setting boundaries don't let others make you feel guilty. Understand selfcare is a necessity and a congruent part of your overall wellbeing. Never under estimate what you can get through with selfcare and balance. And with help from those you know and trust to be there for you. Balance is key.

When I first moved in, to take care of my mother fulltime. It was very difficult for me to balance my time caring for her. 24-hours a day was a lot of for work for me. It had gotten to the place when I left the house to go grocery shopping or to run errands. I would have anxiety attacks and began to rush back home in fear something bad happened. I didn't view taking care of her as job, so I felt guilty leaving her or taking breaks. I was out of balance and I had to learn to rest, take breaks and realize if I didn't, I would be no good to her or myself.

Time is the one thing that we can lose very easily. Therefore, take time to enjoy the season you are in. Take time to smell the "flower", so to speak. Take time to take coffee and tea breaks. And most importantly take time to be grateful for life. Before you know it, you'll wake up one day and learn that you may have missed out on living and enjoying it. Nothing last forever, take advantage of every quiet time and alone time you get.

NOTE: Taking breaks during the day is a good thing. Don't ever feel guilty for taking breaks. When time permits, take a power nap. Taking a nap for 10-20 minutes a day really helps when feeling overwhelmed and anxious.

Taking time away from the day-to-day duties is a must if you want to remain effective. The mind needs quiet time alone. Read a book, take a nap, or take a walk. This will help you feel relaxed and give you the stamina to get back at what you were doing before you took time out to rest.

Organize your day so you will have a sense of timing on how you can organize your work and time for yourself. Caregivers provide care in a wide variety of situations. It can be a very difficult task to accomplish, especially when it involves taking care of an elderly parent. This is a role reversal, which many individuals are not prepared for, nor equipped to handle.

At the time of writing this book, many caregivers fall under the category of taking care of the "baby boomer" generation. This is the generation of elderly population that is aging and living longer. Because of this it's been reported that there are millions of caregivers in the United States currently.

Caregivers must learn to cope with every area of their lives as an integral part to their continued wellness and a healthy lifestyle. To do this successfully, the caregiver must maintain a level of mental health, without becoming too emotionally involved. At times this can become difficult to keep one's emotions in check. Because if not you may get to the point of becoming out of balanced and frustrated and emotionally drained. This can interfere with care for self and for the ones you are caring for.

Note: Caregivers should never be too proud or stubborn to seek help, whether it's from a family member, health care organizations, groups, or professional organizations. Caregivers are caring human beings with real feelings and emotions. And being a caregiver does not exempt one from needing emotional support and help.

CHAPTER VI
SETTING BOUNDARIES

Setting boundaries can be one of the hardest things for caregivers to do. Most caregivers are people pleasers, therefore, many experience compassion fatigue because they are caring. Learning compassion resilience is one skill that allows one to listen to their body. Setting boundaries helps one get renewed by the promptings of their mind, body, spirit, and soul. And if you want to remain healthy and live a long healthy life, you must set boundaries for yourself.

Every adult human being must learn to set boundaries for themselves and not feel guilty for setting them. Caring for others and take a toll on you. Day to day caregiving responsibilities can be overwhelming on you mentally and physically. Learn when to say *no* and when to say yes!

Learning to say no or not now to family, friends and those on the job is a must. Because people are human and they can ask things of you that are outside of your scope as a caregiver. Examples of this would be:

- Loaning money to people you know very well are

unable and unwilling to pay you back.

- Running errands for people that can do it themselves.
- Taking care of people that are physically able to care for themselves.

NOTE: Learn to only do things the person you are caring for cannot do for themselves. You don't want to get burned-out. If they are able to do somethings for themselves then let them do what they can.

Some goals are attainable and some are not when it comes to administering care. You may be able to get the person you are caring for to do certain things for themselves and then you may not. However, don't force the issue and learn to take things in stride. You never want to get frustrated and do things irrational.

Many of you with small children can probably relate. When caring for them try to do things in phases until the goal is accomplished. But never go outside your boundaries trying to make the inevitable, evitable.

Taking care of someone 24 hours a day, can be truly tiresome. However, you have to tell yourself to set limits and boundaries so you can rest and recuperate. Seven days a week, 24 hours a day is hefty. Nevertheless, the work must get done.

If your anything like me, "a workaholic". Then you know you must set boundaries for yourself when it comes to the workload. Along with being a workaholic, I like things organized, neat, and clean. I love to keep those that I care for tidy and clean. So, you have to set boundaries to what you can and cannot do. Somethings like talking on the telephone or watching television all the time may have to decrease.

Learn to take vacations and holidays away from the person you are caring for. Learn to spend time doing things you like to do. And don't become so angry to the point that you fuss over the little trivial things. Set boundaries for yourself and tell yourself, that you can do all things through Christ who strengthens you (Philippians 4:13). Try not to get frustrated to the point you forget somethings can be held off doing at a later date. Don't get to the point where you are so upset, because you can't do all things all the time. Nor is it wise to try to please everybody all the time. Teach people to respect your boundaries so you won't have a mental, emotional, or physical breakdown.

Let's Pause, Break, and Reflect on Your Journey of Caregiving!

Never feel guilting for taking a break and taking care of yourself! Jot down some of the things you want to accomplish within the next six months to a year!

_____

_____

_____

_____

_____

_____

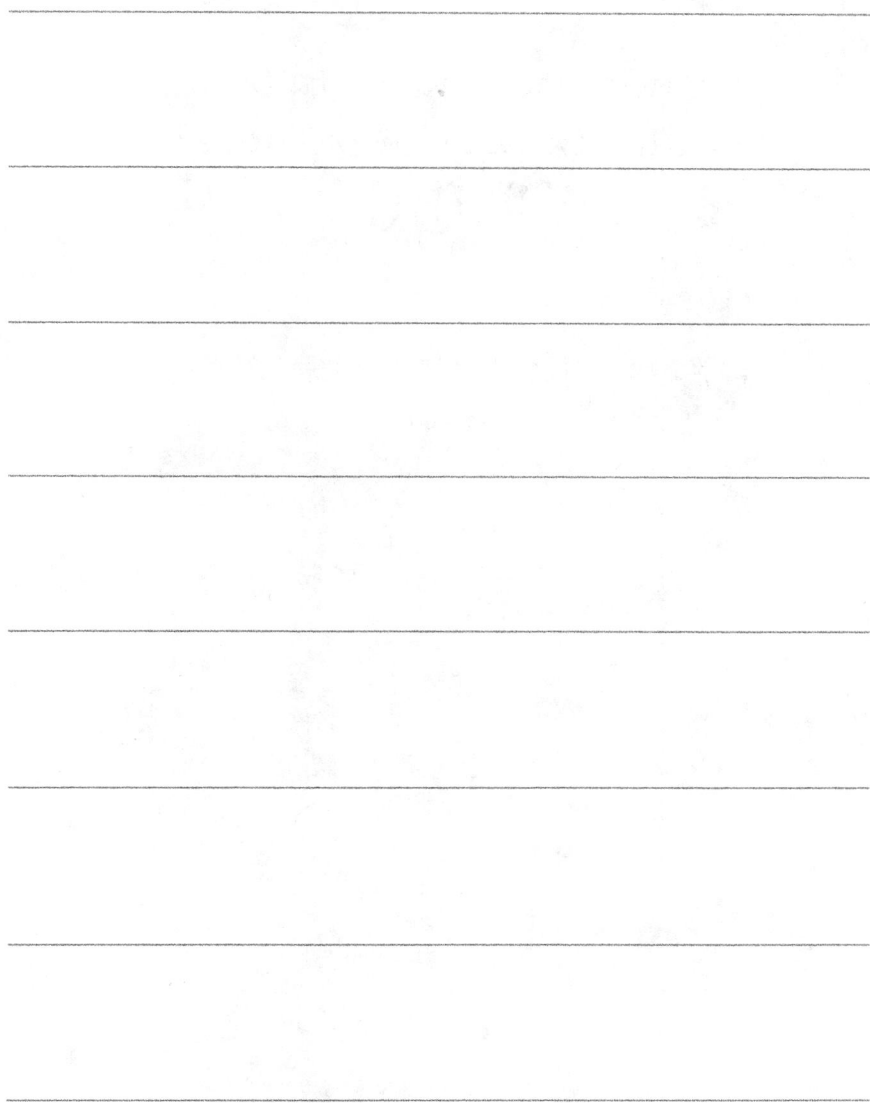

If life hands you lemons, take them and
turn them into lemonade!

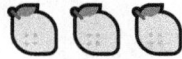

#NoToTheVictimMentality

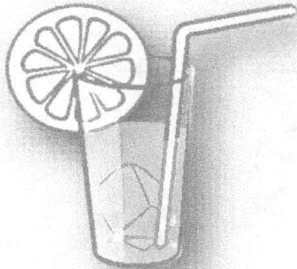

Come unto me, all ye that labor and are heavy laden, and I will give you rest. Take my yoke upon you and learn of me; for I am meek and lowly in heart: and ye shall find rest unto your souls.

Matthew 11:28-29

BEING A CAREGIVER CAN BE OVER
WHELMING.... THIS IS WHY IT'S
IMPERATIVE YOU TAKE TIME TO REST!

And ....
Don't let pride be a hindrance
To you receiving help!

CHAPTER VII
HELP! WHAT ABOUT ME?

It's easy to become frustrated, tired, fatigued, and overwhelmed, when administering care on a daily basis. Taking care of another human being can be a tremendous responsibility. Therefore, you must do somethings to take care of yourself on a daily basis. You can't afford *not* to take care of yourself.

For example, let's look at the analogy of a flight attendant working for a major airline. Before every flight, the flight attendants get in the aisles of the aircraft to perform a safety demonstration. Their announcement - *demonstration* is to inform all passengers in the event of an emergency or loss of cabin oxygen; an oxygen mask will fall from above each passenger's seat. The flight attendant goes on to say each passenger must put their oxygen mask on *first*, before assisting anyone else with their mask. Point is! Take care and save yourself first, so you'll be able to help save someone else's life.

If you are a parent traveling with a small child. The point still remains, put your mask on first. As a parent you'll want to save your child. But you must save yourself first in order to save the child.

Note: The save yourself first concept pertains to all caregivers. Especially caregivers rendering one on one care. Most likely caregivers working in facilities have other caregivers they can rely and call upon. Caregivers that are live-in and homebound don't necessarily have help to assist them with whom they are caring for. Self-care and maintaining good health, is of the essence whomever you are.

You are important and you matter. Without *you* the life that you are caring for may or may not get the proper care. As a caregiver know how important your job is. If you need help, there are different types of resources available to you. In the event you need time to take a break and rest. Please seek the proper help you may need. Such as:

- Hire a sitter.
- Hire a Nurse Assistant or Aide to help you.
- Respite care facilities.

Prepare a list of things that need to be done. The list might include running errands and light housework. Hire someone if you can to sit with your loved ones so you can get out to take care of things you need to get done. Seek solace and rest when you can and let the *helper* choose what she or he can assist you in doing.

Be prepared for hesitancy or refusal. This can be upsetting for the caregiver when a person is unable or unwilling to help. But in the long run, it will do more harm to the relationship if the person helps only because he or she doesn't want to upset you. To the person who seems hesitant, simply say, "Why don't you think about it." Try not to take it personally when a request is turned down. The person is turning down the task, not you. Try not to let a refusal prevent you from asking for help again. The person who refused to help today may be happy to help assist at another time.

Avoid weakening your request. "It's only a thought, but would you consider staying with grandma while I go to church?" This request sounds like it's not very important to you. But going to church may be what you need in order to render care to your grandma. Make specific requests such as: "I would like to go to church on Sunday. Would you stay with grandma from nine a.m. until noon?"

While caregivers will discuss their loved one's care with a physician. Caregivers seldom talk about their own health, which is as vitally important. You matter! Therefore, build a partnership with a physician that addresses your health care needs as well as the recipients needs you are caring for. Hopefully, this partnership can be shared between you, the physician, and other healthcare professionals. This will often require you being assertive, and using good communication skills, to ensure everyone's needs are met—including your own.

NOTE: Here are a few goals and steps to help prevent burnout:

➢ Write down what you need and what you need to do for yourself.
➢ Learn to take breaks from caregiving and get help with caregiving tasks.
➢ Learn to engage in activities that will make you feel healthier.
➢ Make reasonable goals.
➢ Take it slow and don't work on all goals, all at once.
➢ Start off with small steps when planning. Decide which steps you will take first, then get started.

Take a Moment and Jot-Down Some Personal Goals for Yourself!

Care Givers, No Matter How Busy
Or Preoccupied You Become when Caring
for Someone . . . Always Remember to do
Something for Yourself Every day!

#TakeCareOfTheCaregiver

Chapter VIII
The Benefits of Caring for Others

As "baby boomers" age it's going to put a demand on nursing homes and healthcare facilities. Therefore, if you choose to take care of your aging love one at home, you'll need resources and information to help you navigate good care. I have over 20 years of "nursing" and caregiving experience, yet it never ceases to amaze me how much a responsibility it is caring for another!

One of the benefits of caring for others is you reap what you sow. If you have sown good to others, God will make sure you reap good. I know many of you want a financial reward. And the laborer is worthy of his or her hire (work). However, the benefits are more than just mere money. Some of the benefits can be extremely rewarding.

Caregivers are in great demand and you probably know there are lots of opportunities and jobs within most communities. If you enjoy working with people and like having one-on-one interaction with others. Then being a caregiver is for you. If you enjoy taking care of elder family members and like helping others, then you realize the benefit. If you are a caregiver by choice, it's because you chose to be a caregiver or you feel you're the one who can get the job done. Some of the benefits for you are:

- You like working to make a difference in someone's life.
- You like doing a variety of tasks in a day.
- You don't ever say, "that's not my job" but instead like pitching in to do whatever is needed.
- You like making someone smile and doing little things to make a person's day better.
- You take pride in your attention to detail.
- You don't want a desk job; you like being physical in your job and using your body as well as your brain.
- You are seeking a career with growing opportunities.
- You feel that when you are older, you'd want someone like yourself there to help you if you need help.

Taking care of an aging loved one at home can be demanding and it can sometimes feel like a lonely road. The feelings of being overwhelmed can often set in with feelings of thanklessness. Despite all of this, family caregivers persevere and wake up every day to face new challenges. All because they care.

Caregiving is the ultimate act and sacrifice of love. It is a selfless, generous thing to do. Therefore, it is important to give yourself credit for all the work you do. Realize how important your role is as a caregiver. In times of grief and frustration, it is difficult to imagine how in the world caregiving can be considered a positive experience. If you think a little deeper, you'll find the benefits and rewards are extra nominal.

Providing care for another person is a role, that no courses can provide on how to be good at. There are no textbooks on what to expect. Each situation and each person are different. Somehow, you just have to figure it out as you go along. Learn everything you can, get creative and do your best. Caregiving is a huge personal accomplishment, and you should be proud of your resourcefulness, flexibility, and determination.

Even with a difficult patient, caregiving can be one of the most rewarding experiences of your life. It is easy to get wrapped up in the day-to-day grind of providing care. But it's when we adopt this short-sighted perspective, our efforts don't seem very rewarding. Looking back someday, you will probably think that the time you spent with your loved one was incredibly gratifying. When you are feeling overwhelmed, try to take a step back and think about the overall big picture.

One of the biggest fears that people have about illness and death is going through these events alone. Because of you, your loved one will never have to face that. Whether they are of sound mind or struggling with the effects of Dementia, they will understand on some level that you are with them when they need you most. Your time, effort, and attention provide comfort and can have a profound beneficial impact on your loved one. This is a priceless gift.

NOTE: Life is full of ups and downs. When special moments come along that make your heart rejoice. Take a moment and recognition from a loved one's perspective a heartfelt thank you!

Caregiving changes your perspective on life. Looking back on your caregiving journey, you will remember tender moments and highpoints that keep you inspired along the way. Realize what is important to you and what your goals are for yourself, your family, and your own golden years. Even under the most challenging circumstances, taking care of someone you love can have a powerful influence on your outlook, your relationships, and your life.

Never underestimate the impact you have on others. You may not get an award, and you may not even receive any acknowledgment for what you do or what you sacrifice. But always remember you are making a difference in someone's life every day. That's what life is all about.

The decision to help others, show mercy, and to send the message that you are there for them is the ultimate expression of love. It is not easy, but it is commendable. You are part of something bigger than yourself, therefore embrace it.

The essence of life is to serve
others and to do good
~Aristotle

Chapter IX
Expectations

Now that you learned to take care of yourself in the mist of caring for another, what do you think of being a caregiver requires? What do you think the expectations of a caregiver is? And how do those expectations incorporate within your selfcare needs?

Expectation can be defined as, the act or the state of expecting; to wait in expectation; the act or state of looking forward or anticipating; an expectant mental attitude; a high pitch of expectation; something expected; a thing looked forward to. Often expectation is a prospect of future good or profit.

To have great expectations the caregiver must take into consideration that the probability of something happening in relationship to his or her own individual needs will occur. Life happens and expectations are real. A false expectation, is something you may have to take into consideration as well.

False expectations can mean a lot of things to different types of caregivers. The things listed within this chapter of "expectations" are to be considered within the constraints of *false* expectations for caregivers who render in home assistance and those who are live in caregivers. However, note there are other areas caregivers can take consideration to in this list.

False expectations can be:

- You believe or think you can be all things to all people.
- You may still believe that you will be able to enjoy *all* the same freedoms that you had before becoming a caregiver.
- You may believe that you can do, go, and be who you were before you became a caregiver.

Well-meaning people may not understand your true and pure expectations to why you do what you do. As you learn to manage your life and take care of yourself you will find, some people may have to take a back seat in your life. This is not to say that your husband or children will have to. However, some of the things and friends that you were used to may have too.

As you learn to adjust and maintain the flow of things. Things will get better and you will be able to do some of the things like before. But your priority should be to your mental and physical well-being in this season of your life. Don't let the expectations of others, move you out of your commitment to the one you are taking care of. Your expectations should be based on you, your family, and the one you are caring for.

If you are going to practice selfcare then what are your expectations and what are your goals to maintaining maximum health and wellbeing? Are you looking forward to getting out of debt, writing a book, going on a vacation, getting a physical, pedicure and manicure, eating right, etc.?

Note: What expectations to you have in mind? Life goes by quickly. Therefore, plan for something greater. And expect something good to happen in your life.

Just because you are in this season of your life. You do not have to have low expectations. But you must have realistic and attainable goals. Where are you when it comes to caring for yourself? You can be an excellent caregiver. But remember you can get weary sometimes.

Expect to feel overwhelmed sometimes. This is normal. Especially if you are anything like me. Before taking care of my mother. I was so used to being on my own, going when and where I wanted to. And doing what I wanted to. I had to come to the realization that I could not do some of the things I was used to doing as often, anymore. There were times I was so tired I just wanted to sleep and sleep and sleep. But I couldn't. Because I had to take care of mom, who now requires, 24-hour care. It became so overwhelming to the point, I wanted to put her in a nursing home. Trying to maintain my home, her, me, business, work, other relationships, and life caused me to have anxiety. I had to realize that I had to change my expectations and change my thought pattern as well.

Setting goals or deciding what you would like to accomplish in the next three to six months is important. Expect a brighter and healthier future. Take time to achieve your expectations and goals. Seek solutions to difficult situations. And once you have identified a problem, take action to solve it with a positive attitude. Positive people usually are more effective handling problems and use their positive traits as coping abilities.

Identify problems and look at situations with an open mind. The real problem might not be what you think it is. For example, the problem maybe you think you are tired all the time. When the reality to your problem is your belief system, in thinking that no one can care for your love one like you can. This thinking leads to you having to do everything yourself, which is a set-up for fatigue.

Possible solution is to try a different perspective. Hiring someone else to help you is a good thing. Ask a friend to help. Call other resources and seek out reputable agencies in your area that could provide the type of assistance and care you need.

Select a solution then try it! Evaluate yourself how well your choices worked. Then try a second solution. If your first idea does not work. Don't give up! Sometimes an idea just needs fine-tuning.

Ask friends, family members, and professionals for suggestions. If nothing seems to help, accept that the problem may not be solvable for now. You can revisit it another time. Being able to communicate constructively is one of the most important tools you can have. When you communicate in ways that are clear, assertive, confident, and constructive, you will be heard and get the help and support you need.

Take one day at a time and rest whenever possible. Don't let the negative situations distract you and cause you to miss out on the good things in life. Take breaks and take them often. You'll find it's the little things in life that matter. Little breaks from life worries will cause you to flourish and press pass every test and trail.

CAREGIVING IS THE ULTIMATE ACT
OF LOVE. IT IS A SELFLESS, AND A
GENEROUS THING TO DO . . .

CHAPTER X
RISKS FACTORS

There are many risk factors to consider before making a commitment to become a caregiver. There are many factors one must take into consideration as it relates to family matters and time. If you're already a caregiver. You have to take in consideration what risk factors play an important part in who you are and how you can overcome day to day situations.

It appears, some people just have it "made in the shade", so to speak. The misconception that being a caregiver is an easy domesticated task or job is what some think. However, let's get somethings straight. Nobody has the luxury of having it *"made in the shade"*. When looking at the life of a caregiver, you have to understand it is work and it takes physical and mental energy to make it happen.

One must never forget to take time out of your schedule to smell the roses. Look up and admire the possibilities that you will have to endure some kind of suffering as it pertains to life in general, yet alone as a caregiver. Every man that is born of a woman is of few days and yet full of trouble *(sorrow)* - Job 14:1.

Don't miss understand. You will have good days as well as bad days. There is no perfect life. And most caregivers will go through a series of test and trails to do what they do and to accomplish what they accomplish.

Everyone situation is different. You can look at the glass half full or half empty. But you do not have to suffer unnecessarily. In time you will be able to tell whether you are enjoying life in the midst of tests and trails as you administer care to others. Or are you enjoying your life in spite of the risk factors. This is your life and your testimony. We all should be grateful and enjoy life in every season, and every day as able.

I have witnessed many successful caregivers endure suffering. And although, most people you might come to the conclusion you are blessed to be a caregiver and successful to have job where you are able to work a good work. No matter what kind of work this is. Success is a journey in every aspect of life. Therefore, make sure you choose to be mentally, physically, financially, relationally, spiritually successful! Because the payoff is well worth the work.

Effects of being a caregiving can be overwhelming to one's health and well-being. Too often those caring for others experience negative side effects on their health and well-being. Caregiving spouses often experience mental or emotional strain.

The combination of prolonged stress and the physical demands of caregiving, places you at higher risk for significant health problems as well as an earlier death if you are not careful in taking care of yourself.

Caregivers that are taking care of their parents while simultaneously juggling work and raising adolescent children, may face an increased risk of depression, chronic illness, and a possible decline in quality of life.

But despite these risks, family caregivers of any age are less likely than non-caregivers to practice preventive healthcare and self-care behavior. Regardless of age, sex, and race and ethnicity, caregivers report problems attending to their own health and well-being while managing caregiving responsibilities. They report:

- Sleep deprivation.
- Poor eating habits.
- Failure to exercise.
- Failure to stay in bed when ill.

Family caregivers tend to be at risk for depression and excessive use of alcohol, tobacco, and other drugs. Caregiving can be an emotional roller coaster. On one hand, caring for a family member demonstrates love and commitment and can be a very rewarding personal experience. On the other hand, exhaustion, worry, inadequate resources, and continuous care demands are enormously stressful. Therefore, administer self-care to yourself and administer it often.

CHAPTER XI
LEARNING TO GIVE AND RECEIVE

It behooves you to learn to receive all the help, information, and resources you can. With over 20 years of providing care to others. In my experience it never ceases to amaze me how much of a responsibility it is caring for others. I have learned to give all I can to help the one I'm caring for. In hopes of giving them a better quality of life. However, has is still is taking me a while to learn to receive help in return when needed. By nature, I am a very independent person. I like to work alone. However, when it comes to educational resources, research and getting the necessary information needed. I will take a class or subscribe to continual education and training so that I can be better equipped and knowledgeable. Giving and receiving is what it's all about. Learn to receive help. Help can be in the form of people, resources, finances, mental and physical support, informational help, etc...

Sometimes caregivers know more about a patients' condition then the doctor may know. This is because most caregivers assist and take care of patients on a consistent and or daily basis. This goes for one-on-one care, home care, and nursing facilities. Whoever is with the patient the most on a *non*-diagnosis basis is the one who is the voice and heart for the one who is unable to care for themselves. Therefore, receive all the help and all the resources that you can, so your job can be easier. Thus, helping to preserve your health and wellness.

As you become better equipped with the knowledge and resources you need in order to do your job more effectively. Make it your goal to receive. Giving and receiving is to help you maintain your health. Especially for those administering one on one care in home health care and caregivers working in nursing facilities.

Wondering, when is it going to be your turn to receive? I'd say to you, stay focused with your assignment and continue setting goals that you can accomplish in time. Then put them to work. Don't neglect your dreams and visions. Study to show yourself approved. Live right. Treat people right. However, don't be a doormat or use manipulation to get what you want. Trust God's timing and He will make sure *your turn* is inevitable for all to see.

– See Ecclesiastes 9:11

CHAPTER XII
DON'T FORGET TO ENJOY LIFE

For all you do don't forget to enjoy life. Taking care of someone can be bitter and sweet, so to speak. Therefore, don't forget to have fun. Let go and let God. Go to a movie, on a dinner date. Take time out for a vacation if you can. There are respite facilities that can care for you elderly love ones if need. But, whatever you do, do something you like to do at least once a week. Something of interest to you and away from the daily cares and work as a caregiver.

Life is too short and time can slip away very quickly. This is why you must make the best of every day. To live a life of joy and happiness is a good goal to look forward to everyday. In spite of what you may be dealing with as a caregiver. You must deliberately plan date nights and weekend relaxations.

Take note to:

- Vacation at least once a year.

- Get a massage.

- Join a gym or spa.

- Play games or learn to play tennis or activities such as golf.

- Take walks.

- Meditate on positive words of affirmation.

- Study scriptures on healing, joy, and restoration.

Note if you feel overwhelmed meditate on this scripture:

"Come to me, all you who are weary and burdened, and I will give you rest. Take my yoke upon you and learn from me, for I am gentle and humble in heart, and you will find rest for your souls. For my yoke is easy and my burden is light." Matthew 11:28–3 (King James Bible).

Chapter XIII
Organization & Planning

Excess clutter can cause you to feel helpless. Clutter on the outside often represents clutter on the inside. You need organization and planning in your life when caring for others. Not only is this vital for you. It will help you to become organized and intentional about planning your life out.

There are many stages and seasons in life. Being prepared is an absolute must in order to be successful. Caregivers who love being able to take care of the elderly may began to feel overwhelmed by the scope of your role. Or perhaps your partner or close friend spends a significant amount of their time taking care of a loved one and you see the strain it has on them. Feelings of isolation and frustration, anxiety, and lack of sleep, are all real struggles to caregivers widespread.

When a caregiver takes care of themselves, everyone benefits. There are things you can do and ways that will help you to manage the stress that comes with caregiving; and improve your overall quality of life.

Remember the scenario I gave earlier? When you are flying in an aircraft, and the flight attendants start the safety presentation by telling you to put on your oxygen mask first before helping another? Well, the same thing applies to being a caregiver. Only this time it's not an oxygen mask but a whole lot of human needs that should be attended to when taking care of another person.

For you this might mean exercising in the morning before assuming your caregiving role. Or it could be taking time out to journal each day and organize your thoughts. Whatever it is you like to do to relax and center yourself, make sure you work it into your day. Believe me, your love ones will appreciate the happier, more relaxed version of "you."

Caregiving can take a lot of your time, with little left over for seeing friends or getting out of the house. It might make you feel a little despondent when you are spending a lot of time with a very sick or elderly person and the last thing you feel like doing is going out.

Whatever it is that is holding you back from socializing with people outside of the caregiving bubble, recognize it and work a way around it. Socializing is proven to help reduce stress.

Stress management is one of the most difficult aspects of caregiving. Considering that we are often deal with multiple things at different times of the day, things can get intimidating.

Caregivers have to stay on track and adherence to stay well and physically fit.

Caregiving might seem like hard work, but there are moments in between when you get to spend quality time with the person you are caring for and this can be rewarding.

Depending on the mobility of the person you are looking after, this can range from a short walk or drive in nature, a game of cards, watching a movie together, or simply listening to a story they enjoy telling. While life can seem like a long list of tasks, this role won't continue forever, but these moments can make a world of difference to you both.

Lean on others because there's no way around it. Caregiving can be an incredibly lonely role to play. You may feel isolated, sad, frustrated, exhausted… And on top of it all, you may feel guilty about feeling those things!

Do not underestimate both the physical and emotional toll it can take on you, and make sure to lean on others for support. Grab a coffee with a friend and talk to them about how you feel. Join a support group at your local hospital or nursing home and share and vent with people in a similar situation as yourself. Check out the guide from AARP on caregiver resources in your area.

It may be hard to imagine leaving your loved one in the care of someone else for any period of time, but sometimes it's exactly what you need. Just as a mother of young children needs to get some headspace from time to time in order to come back refreshed and focused in her role as "mom," you will benefit from having some time away from your caregiver role.

There are various options open to you for respite care, ranging from in-home respite (when a health care aide comes to your home to provide nursing services or simply companionship) to short term care nursing homes that can look after your loved one if you take some time off.

Chapter XIV
Rest and Relaxation

Rest and relaxation are very similar but not the same. However, both are vitally important to maintaining your overall health, so you can remain being beneficial to those you care for and administer care to. As we mentioned before caregivers are very driven when it comes to helping others. If you are genuinely a caregiver you will have a tendency to want to put others before your needs. And this can mean at the experience of you needing to say and "no" to what you think is important before you get some needed rest.

Most caregivers are also night owls. Because they usually work throughout the day meeting the needs and demands of the home, the children, and if they are administering care inside the home. They usually are very busy all throughout the day and in some cases throughout the night caring for others.

Therefore, it is imperative that you as a caregiver, don't become so obsessed with staying up late nights or working overtime to compensate time taking care of yourself. Because the best care you can give yourself is rest.

Isaiah 30:15 states, "For thus saith the Lord GOD, the Holy One of Israel; In returning and rest shall ye be saved; in quietness and in confidence shall be your strength: and ye would not." I love this scripture and when I am feeling weary, I turn to it and meditate often when I am feeling overwhelmed or tired. However, notice the later part of this scripture where it states, "but you would not!"

Do not be so full of pride that you refuse to rest. Resting and trusting God to send you help or that He will help you on your caregiving journey when you are feeling overwhelmed and plain ole tired.

Rest can include but is not limited to..........

- Naps
- Breaks
- Quietness
- Sleep
- Mediation
- Non-movement
- Prayer
- Imagery
- Solitude

- Holiday
- Vacation
- Massage
- Reading
- No-Activity

Exercise promotes better sleep, reduces tension and depression, and increases energy and alertness.

CHAPTER XV
HEALTH AND WELLNESS

Now that I think about it, I should have put this chapter in the beginning of the book. Because being healthy and well are very important components of being a caregiver. Being a caregiver is hard work and some doctors think of caregivers as "hidden patients." Studies show that caregivers are much more likely than non-caregivers to suffer from health issues such as, stress overload, depression, anxiety, and other health issues.

Staying healed, healthy, whole, and well in every aspect of your life is the goal. However, many caregivers are over extended, over worked in most cases just plain old tired. Many may not or even consider their overall health and wellbeing. Because caregivers in general get a sense of fulfilment in taking care of others.

Women tend to multitask more so then men. And are prone to be nurtures by instinct. And they tend to be the primary caregivers in society. Nothing is wrong with this. However, ladies we need to take better care of ourselves. In order to be successful at administering care. We must also maintain health and wellness. This is also for male caregivers as well.

It is vital to eat right, think right and live right if you want maintain wholeness and health. There are so many ways to get the proper information. The world wide web is an excellent tool to do your research and to learn how to eat healthy and right!

Always read the food labels. And make sure the foods that you are consuming is good and healthy food. Always drink the proper amounts of fluids and water. And try to avoid taking in excessive amounts of sodas, pops, and sweet sugary drinks. Fruit juices are healthy however that do contain a lot of carbohydrates to be aware of this.

Although I am not a nutritionist and can only advise you so far. There is a lot of information online. Always seek to maintain optimum health. Because if you are not healthy how can you help care for others. It is possible to care for others and you be unhealthy. However, its beneficial that you maintain good health first and for most.

Exercise is particularly important to health and wellness. I love to walk. Therefore, I take brisk walks at least two times a week. One, two, three, miles is healthy for you. Whatever, the form of exercise you like to do. Do it. At all cost be creative with how you plan to work out and exercise if you are home bound and unable to get to a gym or work out facility. For example:

- Taking the stairs
- Jogging in place
- Sit-ups
- Squats
- Stretches
- Stomach Crunches
- Home Exercise DVD's
- Home Workout Equipment:
  - ✓ Treadmills
  - ✓ Bicycles
  - ✓ Take a half-hour break during the week.
  - ✓ Walk three times a week.

You may be reluctant to start exercising, even though you have heard it's one of the healthiest things you can do. Perhaps you think that physical exercise might harm you, or that it is only for people who are young and able to do things like jogging. Fortunately, research suggests that you can maintain or at least partly restore endurance, balance, strength, and flexibility through every day physical activities like walking and gardening. Even household chores can improve your health. The key is to increase your physical activity by exercising and using your own muscle power.

Exercise promotes better sleep, reduces tension and depression, and increases energy and alertness. If finding time for exercise is a problem, incorporate it into your daily activity. Perhaps the care recipient can walk or do stretching exercise with you. If necessary, do frequent short exercises instead of those that require large blocks of time. Find activities you enjoy.

Walking, one of the best and easiest exercises, is a great way to get started. Besides its physical benefits, walking helps to reduce psychological tension:

- Walking twenty minutes a day, three times a week, is greatly beneficial. If you cannot get away for that long, try to walk for as long as you can on however many days you can.
- Work walking into your life.
- Walk around the mall, to the store, or a nearby park.
- Walk around the block with a friend.

Visit and communicate with your physician annually. Prepare questions ahead of time and make a list of your most important concerns and problems. Issues you might want to discuss with the physician are changes in general physical and mental health. Make sure you let him or her know what your concerns are in terms of your daily care and health.

You will have good days as well as bad days! Therefore, Learn to enjoy every day!

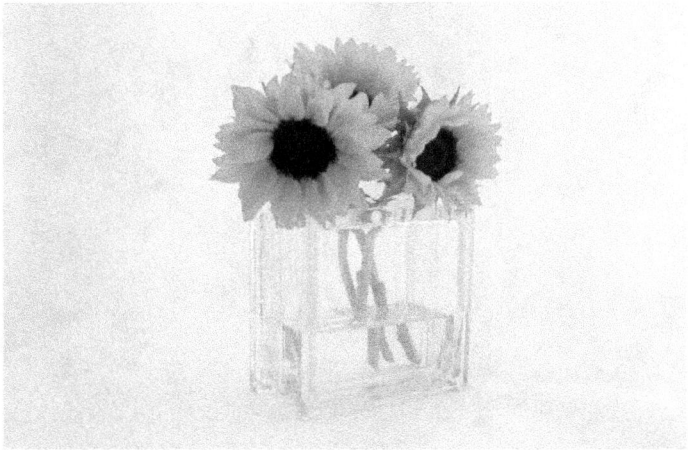

CHAPTER XVI
PRAYER AND MEDITATION

Prayer and meditation are the lifeline for your spiritual wellbeing. There is a much better chance of you becoming a more excellent caregiver that is not frightened by overwhelming circumstances that comes along with being a caregiver. Take a wholeness approach to being whole spiritually, physically, mentally, and financially, through prayer and meditation is a must.

Prayer helps you to say focused and sane. Let's face it there is so much to do and deal with when you are a caregiver. Being a caregiver is all about taking care of another human being. Therefore, you want to make sure you are prayed up and ready for the task daily.

Some might say what if I don't know how to pray? Well let me help you to understand. Prayer is very simple yet profound. Praying with your mouth, heart and soul is simply talking to God. Telling Him all about your cares, problems, and wants. God is concerned about everything that goes on in your life. By the way of prayer, you can talk to God and communicate to Him, what you need to accomplish in every task. Even though God already knows what you have need of. For some reason He loves to hear from His creation.

Meditate on positive things and the word of God also known as the *bible*. When referring to the bible, the scriptures contain the answers to life. For in the bible is the breath and life of God. Everything you have need of is in the book. It may or may not be in a tailored translation to your specific problem. However, what the word of God has to say will line up with every situation, whether it's good or bad. Every situation has an answer. If you need help on how to treat people, it's in the bible. If you need help on how to manage your time and resources, it's in the bible. If you need help on how to treat yourself it's in the bible. Meditate and apply the scriptures along with all the practical knowledge you have on being a caregiver.

NOTE: Use this book as a positive reference, reinforcement, and encouragement along with the bible and other resources to help you get throughout your caregiving journey.

In life test and trials come to teach and help us get to the

next level in dealing with people and things that pertain to

our caregiving experiences. If we learn to turn tests and

trails into opportunities we can and will have success.

GOD IS JUST A PRAYER AWAY! HE
IS WAITING TO GIVE YOU PEACE
AND ANSWERS TO WHATEVER
AILS YOU!

HAVE A TALK WITH JESUS
EVERYDAY!

Serenity Prayer
God grant me the serenity to accept
the things I cannot change,
Courage to change the things I can,
and wisdom to know the difference.

Prayer Notes

Appendix 1

Reflections

Peace in the mist of the storm. Let's talk about how going through the storms of life.

Not every storm is designed to kill you! Sometimes the storm is designed to make you better and take you to another level.

- Better Not Bitter!
- Better NOT Forsaken!
- Better NOT Forgotten!

Matthew 14:22-33King James Version (KJV) says,

> And straightway Jesus constrained his disciples to get into a ship, and to go before him unto the other side, while he sent the multitudes away. And when he had sent the multitudes away, he went up into a mountain apart to pray: and when the evening was come, he was there alone. But the ship was now in the midst of the sea, tossed with waves: for the wind was contrary.

And in the fourth watch of the night Jesus went unto them, walking on the sea. And when the disciples saw him walking on the sea, they were troubled, saying, it is a spirit; and they cried out for fear. But straightway Jesus spoke unto them, saying, be of good cheer; it is I; be not afraid. And Peter answered him and said, Lord, if it be, thou, bid me come unto thee on the water. And he said, Come. And when Peter was come down out of the ship, he walked on the water, to go to Jesus. But when he saw the wind boisterous, he was afraid; and beginning to sink, he cried, saying, Lord, save me. And immediately Jesus stretched forth his hand, and caught him, and said unto him, O thou of little faith, wherefore didst thou doubt? And when they were come into the ship, the wind ceased. Then they that were in the ship came and worshipped him, saying, Of a truth thou art the Son of God.

II

*Let's talk about being weary and praising God,
even when you don't feel like it.*

Praising God in the midst of being tired, frustrated, and weary is an
excellent opportunity to get the strength you may need at the appointed
time. To be honest it is one of the best times to give God praise. Praise
God when you need help, a miracle, a blessing, or financial break
through. Storms and the trails of life are some of the perfect times to
praise and to pray.

This is why I ask you to take time out of your day. Every day to reflect
on the positive things and not he the situation. Praise God and thank Him
every day even when you don't feel like it. Because if the truth be told
someone is always worst off then yourself. And there is always someone
that would love to take your place in retrospect of the good things that
are happening in your circumstances as a caregiver.

It is a very demanding job or assessment to being a caregiver. Whether
you are in the home, someone else's home or working as a caregiver.
However, expect God to bless you and expect Him to move or your
behalf. Because how many of know that it's time to see God move
especially in social, economic times like these. These are the days when
God wants to perform miracles!

III

In order to get to the next level, you have to go through test and trials.

Mark 4:38-40 states, Jesus Himself was in the stern, asleep on the cushion; and they woke Him and said to Him, "Teacher, do You not care that we are perishing?" And He got up and rebuked the wind and said to the sea, "Hush, be still." And the wind died down and it became perfectly calm. And He said to them, "Why are you afraid? Do you still have no faith?"

Ephesians 5:20-21 states; God is able to do exceedingly and abundantly all that we can think or image. Now to Him who is able to do far more abundantly beyond all that we ask or think, according to the power that works within us, to Him be the glory in the church and in Christ Jesus to all generations forever and ever. Amen.

- Storms come to make you better and to set you up for a miracle, a healing, a financial breakthrough or whatever it is you have need of.

- In the midst of a storm is the perfect time to turn to God and to lean and trust in Him.

- The devil comes to scare you and to tell you God is not concerned. However, in most cases God is right there with you in the storm. Just waiting on you to control of your situation.

- Some storms require immediate attention

- Others require you to just ride them out

- There are some storms that require you to take cover.

James 1:12 English Standard Version (ESV)

Blessed is the man who remains steadfast under trial,

for when he has stood the test, he will receive the crown

of life, which God has promised to those who love him.

Appendix II

Scriptures

These scriptures are easy to memorize and they will help you stay
focused and help you keep your mind and heart at peace when
the stress of caregiving gets to an overwhelming stage.

Come to Me, all you who labor and are heavy laden, and I will give you
rest. Matthew 11:28

Whatever you do, work at it with all your heart, as working for the Lord, not for
human masters.... It is the Lord Christ you are serving. Colossians 3:23–24

I believe that I shall look upon the goodness of the LORD in the land of the
living! Wait for the LORD; be strong, and let your heart take courage; wait for
the LORD! Psalm 27:13-14

Do not fear, for I am with you; do not be dismayed, for I am your God. I will
strengthen you; I will help you, yes, I will uphold you with My righteous right
hand. Isaiah 41:10

Blessed be God, the Father of our Lord Jesus Christ, the Father of mercies, and the God of all comfort, who comforts us in all our tribulation, that we may be able to comfort those who are in any trouble by the comfort with which we ourselves are comforted by God. 2 Corinthians 1:3-4

Yea, though I walk through the valley of the shadow of death, I will fear no evil; for You are with me; Your rod and Your staff, they comfort me. Psalm 23:4

Trust in the Lord with all your heart and lean not on your own understanding; in all your ways submit to him, and he will make your paths straight. Proverbs 3:5–6

Cast all your anxiety on him because he cares for you. I Peter 5:7

DOCUMENT CAREGIVING EXPERIENCES!

_____

_____

_____

_____

_____

_____

About the Author

Christine is a servant leader at heart, with a desire to help people mature in their giftings and callings. She has over 20 years' experience in nursing as a Caregiver, Home Health Aide, Certified Nurse Assistant (CNA), Medical Assistant, and a host of student nursing (SN) credit hours.

She attended University of Detroit Mercy Nursing School for several years. However, she resigned from nursing school to pursue a Masters in Non-profit Management and a Doctorate in Ministry (D. Min). She current takes care of her mother; and serves in various outreaches via social media and ministers to those throughout her community.

She has authored and published several books and looks forward to fulling her God given assignment by helping those in need.

Other Books by Author:

The Happy Life Style

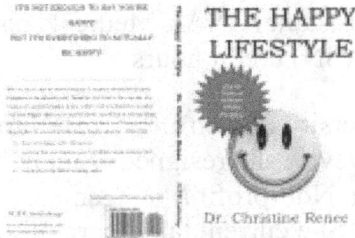

The Harvest: Preparing the Labors for the End Times

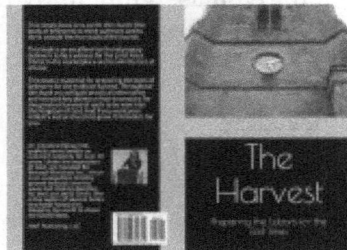

Taking Care of the Caregiver

Christine Renee

For more information about the author, books and
speaking seminars contact Christine Renee at:

HAR Publishing
USA

www.HARPublishing.com

www.ingramcontent.com/pod-product-compliance
Lightning Source LLC
Chambersburg PA
CBHW060506280326
41933CB00014B/2884